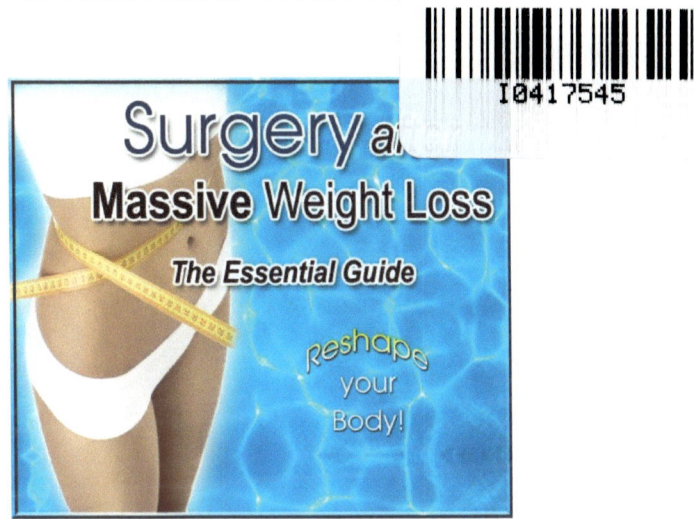

Copyright ©2010 by Dr. Anire Okpaku, MD, FACS

Printed in the United States of America

ISBN: 145154555X

SURGERY AFTER MASSIVE WEIGHT LOSS

The Essential Consumer Guide

By Dr. Anire Okpaku, MD, FACS

Dr. Anire Okpaku MD, FACS

1900 Brickell Avenue
Miami, FL 33129

CALL US: 305.856.9566 »

TABLE OF CONTENTS

Introduction

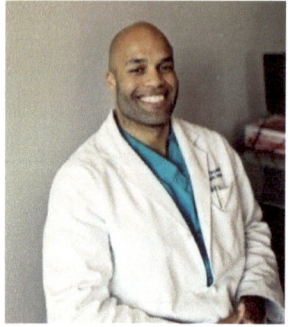

"Thank you for your interest in our services and for ordering this guide. I hope this information helps you learn more about our procedures and to inform you about what to expect with weight loss and surgery. If you have more questions please do not hesitate to call my office and schedule a consultation with me, my door is always open."

-- Dr. Anire Okpaku, MD, FACS

The Benefits Of Weight Loss

Losing weight will improve your health, stamina, and mental disposition in many ways. Just losing a small amount of your current weight can make a difference in the way you feel and look. Here are some other ways weight loss can benefit your health:

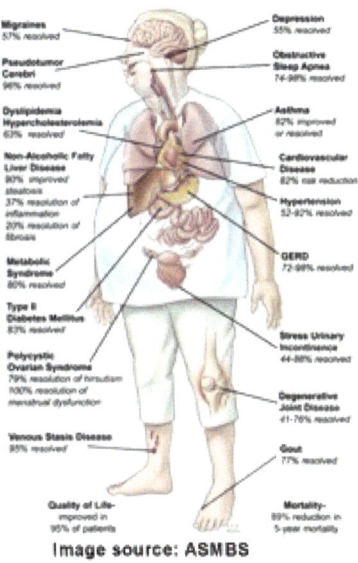

Image source: ASMBS

- Increased energy level
- Lowered cholesterol levels
- Reduced blood pressure
- Reduced aches and pains
- Improved mobility
- Improved breathing
- Helps you sleep better and wake up more rested
- Prevention of angina chest pain caused by decreased oxygen to the heart
- Decreases your risk of sudden death from heart disease or stroke
- Prevention of Type 2 diabetes
- Improvement of blood sugar levels

Combating Obesity:

According to federal statistics, nearly a third (30 percent) of adult Americans are now obese and over 5 percent are morbidly or severely obese. Today there are choices to combat obesity which can lead to dramatic weight loss:

- Proper nutrition/Change of diet
- Exercise
- Bariatric Surgery (Gastric Bypass/Lap band)
- Other forms of medical treatments

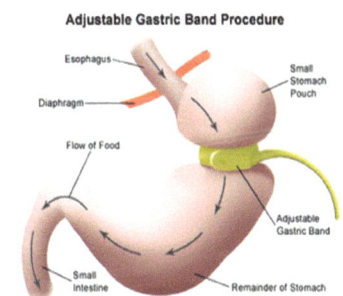

Adjustable Gastric Band Procedure

Why Surgery After Massive Weight Loss?

Once you reach your weight loss goals you may find you do not have the fit and healthy body image you expected. After massive weight loss, the skin and tissues that have been severely stretched over the years, lack elasticity and cannot readjust to the new, smaller size of the body. As a result, sagging pockets of skin may form around the face, neck and jaw line, at the upper arms, lower back, the abdomen region and around the hips, buttocks, groin area and thighs.

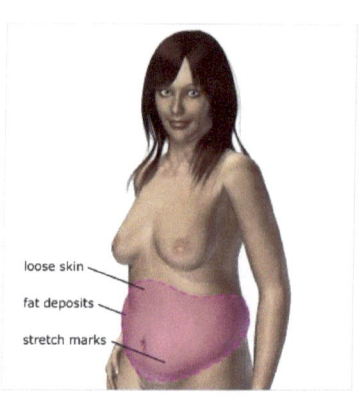

loose skin

fat deposits

stretch marks

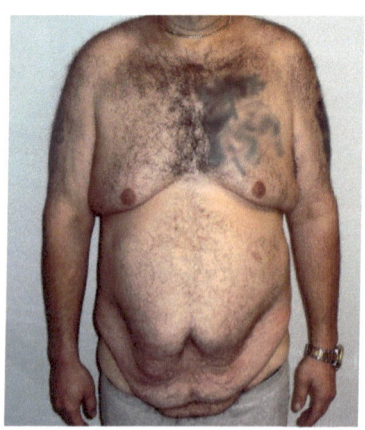

The surplus, sagging skin that is left behind after massive weight loss, can cause considerable hygienic problems, skin irritation, skin breakdown, pain and even infection. This loose, sagging skin looks abnormal in most cases and gets in the way of normal activities or movement.

Aging, pregnancy, some genetic skin conditions, and major weight loss can also result in severe hanging tissues, considering the body is a three dimensional object. When the problem extends around the body, Body Lift Surgery can address loose drooping tissues all around the body. Body Lift Surgery often involves several stages to address the entire body: Lower Body Lift, Breast Lift, Arm Lift, Thigh Lift, Upper Body Lift among other procedures.

Trends:

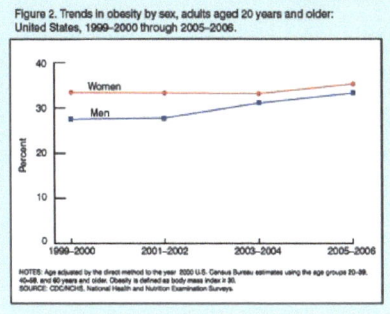

Figure 2. Trends in obesity by sex, adults aged 20 years and older: United States, 1999–2000 through 2005–2006.

NOTES: Age adjusted by the direct method to the year 2000 U.S. Census Bureau estimates using the age groups 20–39, 40–59, and 60 years and older. Obesity is defined as body mass index ≥ 30.
SOURCE: CDC/NCHS, National Health and Nutrition Examination Surveys.

Latest estimates[1] indicate that in 2005 alone, U.S. plastic surgeons performed nearly 56,000 post-operative body-contouring procedures on patients who had undergone bariatric surgery.

For over 170,000 morbidly obese patients who undergo the surgery each year in the United States, this procedure is just the first step back to health and a positive self-esteem.

One surgical option is a series of operations called body contouring, where Dr. Okpaku removes the excess tissue, sculpts and restores the body to a more normal, aesthetically pleasing state, and for most patients this is a positive transformation, a dramatic return to health and self-confidence.

These state of the art procedures such as Dr. Okpaku's Total Body Lift™ , Corset Trunkplasty, Abdominoplasty, Panniculectomy and more, are just some of the new cutting edge techniques skillfully performed by Dr. Okpaku to safely restore normalcy and self-confidence to his grateful patients after massive weight loss.

1. *Medical News Today, Nov 2006*

COMMON POST BARIATRIC SURGICAL PROCEDURES:

Breasts

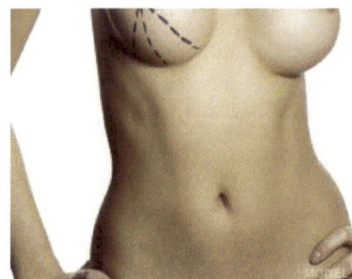

Dr. Okpaku believes all women want to look and feel beautiful. Cosmetic breast enhancement enables women to make lasting changes to their looks so they can regain confidence in their image and feel comfortable in their body. The size and shape of a woman's breasts can often play a critical role in a woman's self image.

Women who are discontent with their breast size can often feel self-conscious or even embarrassed about their appearance. We offer a variety of breast enhancement procedures that will give the breasts a more balanced, symmetrical look while still appearing natural and beautiful.

Breast Lift

A breast lift will raise and firm sagging, flat breasts. Some patients also may require breast implants to improve the shape and size. Incisions are placed around the nipple, from the nipple to the crease under the breast, and sometimes horizontally along the breast crease.

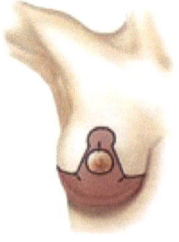
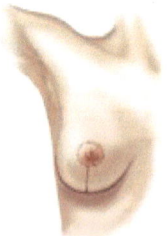

Recovery Process

Generally, post-operative instructions call for plenty of rest and limited movement in order to speed up the healing process and reduce the recovery time. Bandages are applied immediately following surgery to aid the healing process and to minimize movement of the breasts. Once the bandages are removed, a specialized surgical bra will need to be worn for several weeks. Patients sometimes report minor pain associated with surgery. Any pain can be treated with oral medication. While complications are rare, patients can minimize potential problems by carefully following the instructions given after surgery.

Breast Reduction

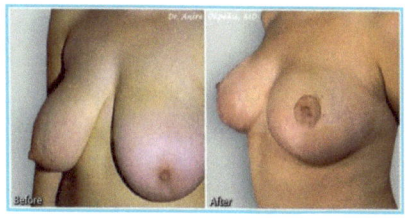

Breast reduction (or reduction mammoplasty) is an enhancement procedure that reshapes the breasts in order to make them smaller, lighter, and firmer. Reduction is accomplished by removing excess fat, glandular tissue, and skin. Large breasts can cause physical pain as well as emotional and social anxiety. Women who take advantage of the breast reduction procedure find that they are able to lead a healthier, more comfortable life, in addition to enjoying a beautiful, more proportionate appearance.

Reasons for Considering a Breast Reduction:
• Back, neck or shoulder pain caused by heavy breasts.
• Sagging breasts produced by their large size.
• Disproportionate body frame attributed to oversized breasts.
• Restriction of physical activity due to the size and weight of the breasts.
• Painful bra strap marks and/or rashes as a result of large breasts.

General Procedure

Techniques for breast reduction vary; however, the most common procedure involves an incision that circles the areola. From the areola, the incision goes down and follows the natural curve under the breast. The surgeon then removes excess glandular tissue, fat, and skin. Next, the nipple and areola are repositioned to a higher position and held in place by stitches. Other methods include a vertical mastopexy where the

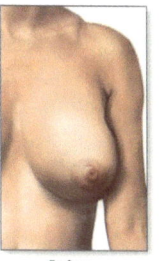

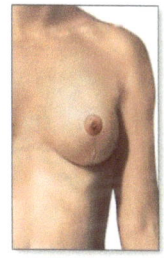

Before   After healing

insicion goes around the nipple and down (Lollipop Lift). Occasionally, liposuction alone can be used to reduce breast size. The best procedure can be determined during the initial consultation visit. Of all plastic surgery procedures, breast reduction results in the quickest body-image changes. Patients are pleased with the elimination of physical pain caused by large breasts as well as a better proportioned body, an enhanced appearance, and better fitting clothes.

Breast Augmentation

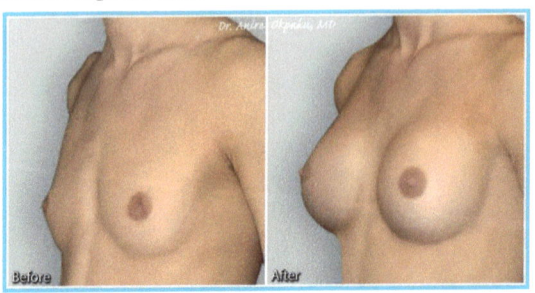

Breast augmentation, also known as mammoplasty, is a surgical enhancement procedure to accentuate the size and shape of a woman's breasts. While breast augmentation will make the breasts larger, the surgery will not move the breasts closer together or lift sagging breasts. Breast augmentation is tremendous help to patients who desire a fuller profile, who have lost breast volume due to pregnancy or nursing, or who have undergone breast reconstruction and want to gain a more natural look again.

Reasons for Considering Breast Augmentation:

• Enhance body shape if breasts are too small.
• Increase breast volume after pregnancy and nursing.
• Equalize a difference in breast size (cup size) to gain breast symmetry.
• Reconstruct breasts following a mastectomy or injury. General Procedure

Breast augmentation involves making a small incision to insert a breast implant into the breast area in order to enlarge the breast. The surgery is commonly performed on an outpatient basis at a hospital or state-of-the-art surgical unit while the patient is under a general anesthesia and asleep. There are several possible locations for the small incision that will be used for inserting the breast implant. A common technique utilizes an incision made in the lower portion of the breast. Another technique, though less frequently used, involves making an incision in the armpit. Dr. Okpaku's preferred technique is making an inferior areola incision. The best technique will be decided together between the patient and the surgeon during the consultation.

During surgery, the breast tissue is raised to create an open pocket under the breast tissue or beneath the chest wall muscle. Inserting an implant behind each breast can increase a woman's breast size by one or more bra cup sizes. Implants typically contain a saline solution (similar to saltwater) or silicone gel, both of these types of implants are FDA cleared for cosmetic surgery. In some circumstances, particularly those in which there is breast asymmetry (uneven breast size), an inflatable implant may be used to allow the surgeon to adjust the level of inflation to attain breast symmetry and balance. Surgery typically takes about one hour.

Male Pectoral Implants

There have been increases in the number of men who want to enhance their bodies through cosmetic surgery. Many men who can't achieve their desired results from working out or can't find the time to make it to the gym rely on pectoral implant surgery to enhance the appearance of their bodies.

Others undergo the procedure to correct both congenital and physical defects. One of the most popular procedures today among men, pectoral implants are used to shape, enlarge, and firm the upper chest.

Overview

Male pectoral implants are made of silicone and are placed underneath the pectoral muscles. Unlike female breast implants, which are filled with liquid, the male silicone implant is soft, but solid. Pec implant surgery is usually done on an outpatient basis. The patient will be allowed to go home after the surgery following strict instructions from their surgeons. Depending on one's body, the healing process can take as long as six weeks.

Risks and Complications

Like any other surgeries, getting male pec implants may pose certain risks. Complications may include the displacement of the implants, infections, hematoma, seroma, and numbness of the inner upper arm.

Due to the stress placed on the pectoral muscles during everyday activities, there is a likelihood that the implant will shift after surgery.

Medial Thigh Lift

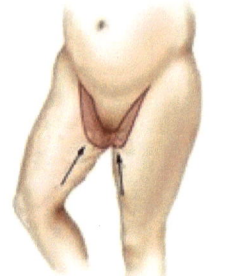 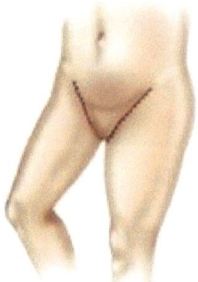

The medial thigh lift will lift and tighten the sagging skin of the inner thigh. Incisions are usually placed in the groin.

Panniculectomy

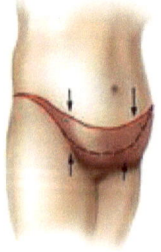 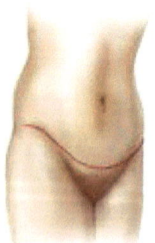

A panniculectomy is performed to remove the hanging pannus, or apron of skin, from the lower abdomen below the belly button. The excess skin and fat above the belly button are not removed. A panniculectomy is often performed on patients who are still significantly overweight but have skin irritation from their hanging skin. After surgery, these patients have less skin problems but have little improvement in the contour of their bellies.

Abdominoplasty (Tummy Tuck)

A tummy tuck, or abdominoplasty, is one of the most common cosmetic surgery procedures performed. Often, factors such as multiple pregnancies and genetics can contribute to the development of loose skin, fat deposits, and stretch marks in the abdominal region. Even substantial weight loss can contribute to the development of loose skin in the abdomen. As these areas typically persist despite proper diet and exercise, they can make the abdomen appear disproportionate with the rest of the body.

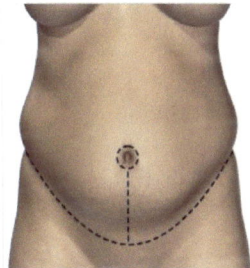

An Abdominoplasty requires a horizontal incision in the area between the navel and the public bone. The length of the incision is to be determined by the amount of correction necessary to achieve your goals and more specifically the amount of skin to be reduced. The incision may be only a few inches in length, may extend from hip to hip or may extend beyond the hip to achieve optimal results.

A second incision around the navel may be necessary to correct excess skin in the upper abdomen. Through the incision, weaken abdominal muscles will be repaired, if necessary. Excess fat will be removed using surgically or liposuction techniques and excess tissue and skin will be removed. Your incision will be closed with sutures or surgical clips.

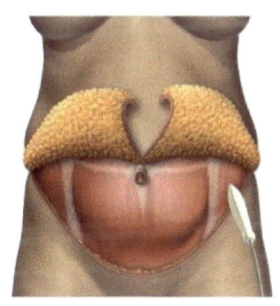

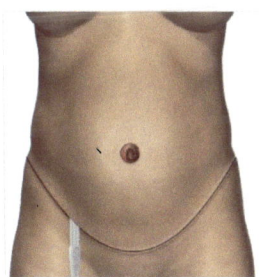

Following your Tummy Tuck you may have small thin tubes placed in your incisions to drain any excess fluid that accumulates or you may be placed in a compression garment or wrap in elastic bandages to reduce swelling,

How a Full Tummy Tuck Works

A full tummy tuck works by removing loose skin, fat deposits, and stretch marks from the abdominal region. In addition, vertical abdominal muscles that have been stretched and weakened over time are tightened, restoring the appearance of a firmer, flatter abdomen. Tummy tuck procedures can be performed alone, but are often performed with liposuction to further improve

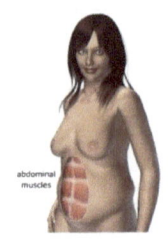

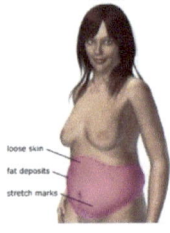

body contours. A tummy tuck should not be considered as a treatment for obesity, or a substitute for proper diet and exercise. Individuals considering a tummy tuck should be healthy and relatively fit. Future pregnancies and substantial changes in weight following a tummy tuck, as well as the presence of scars from prior surgeries may decrease the effectiveness and longevity of treatment.

1-Incision

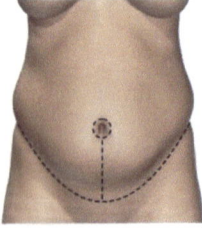

Full tummy tuck procedures typically require two incisions. The surgeon will make an incision just above the pubic area that spans from one hip bone to the other. The length of the incision and its shape will depend on the extent of treatment as well as the contours of your body. While the surgeon will attempt to place the incision so that it is hidden by a bathing suit or undergarments, it is important to realize that you will have a permanent scar. A second incision is usually made around the navel.

2-Exposure of Abdominal Wall

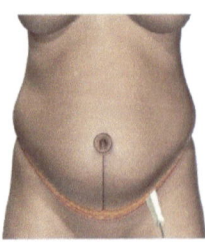

The skin and fat layers that lie above the abdominal wall are separated from the wall using a cautery device. The tissue is then lifted upward toward the rib cage to expose the abdominal muscles.

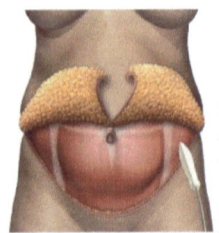

3-Tightening of Abdominal Muscles

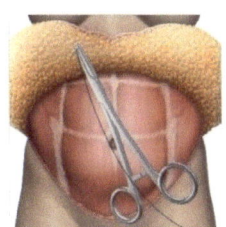

In order to tighten the abdomen, the surgeon will suture the abdominal muscles, pulling them closer together, which creates a flatter, firmer abdominal wall and a slimmer waistline.

4-Replacing Skin and Navel Position

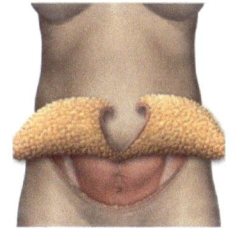

The surgeon will stretch the layer of skin and fat that had been lifted away back tightly over the abdominal wall. Although your navel remains intact and attached to the abdominal wall, it will become covered by the layer of skin when it is pulled back into place. Therefore, the surgeon will make an incision through the layers of skin and fat to create a new hole for your navel. The skin and fat that hangs beyond the original incision line will be removed.

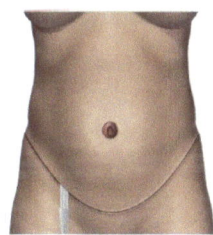

5-Incision Closure

In order to prevent fluid buildup as you heal, drainage tubes will likely be placed in the abdomen, and will remain in place for approximately 3-7 days. The incisions will be sutured and dressings and bandages will be applied.

6-Full Tummy Tuck Recovery

After tummy tuck surgery, you may have to wear a special compression garment, which is similar to a girdle. This tight-fitting garment will help reduce swelling by preventing excessive fluid buildup, as well as providing comfort and will support you as you heal. The length of time required to use the garment will depend on the extent of the surgery. In some cases you may have to wear the girdle up to several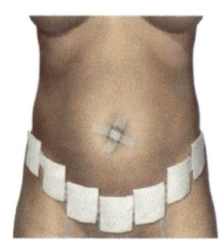
weeks. As with any major surgical procedure, you will likely experience pain, bruising, and swelling, most of which will subside in a few weeks.

While you may not be able to stand fully upright, it is important that you begin to walk for short periods soon after your procedure to facilitate blood flow. Your stitches may dissolve with time. However non-dissolving stitches will be removed in approximately one week.

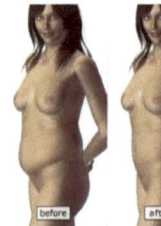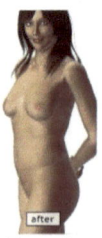

7-Full Tummy Tuck Results

Most patients are able to return to work in one to three weeks time. However, it may take six to eight weeks before you feel able to return to full normal activity including heavy lifting and strenuous exercise. Although you will have a permanent scar, it will slowly fade over time. It is important to realize that if you become pregnant or experience substantial weight gain or loss, the results from your procedure may be compromised. However, with proper diet and exercise, the results from a tummy tuck can be maintained for years.

Who will benefit from a Tummy Tuck Surgery ?

People who lost a lot of weight, which have skin that has not reshaped to the new abdominal contour will benefit most from a tummy tuck. Women that have had children will also benefit since pregnancy does stretch the abdominal skin. A cesarean tends to scar the underlying abdominal wall and leaves some patients with a slight overhand over that scaring.

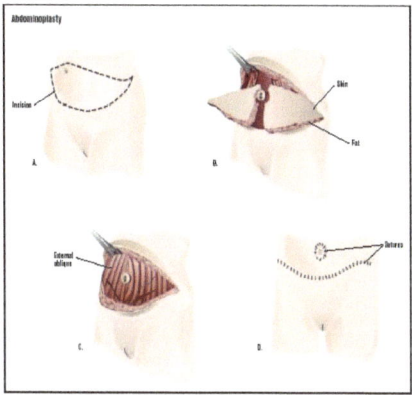

Some things to consider when you are contemplating a Tummy Tuck. First of all, consider the muscles in your tummy. Normally during pregnancy the muscles in your tummy will split a bit. Often in your recovery period from the pregnancy they tend to go back to some extent, they don't always go back fully.   How do you test if you have this condition, known as *diastasis rectus ?

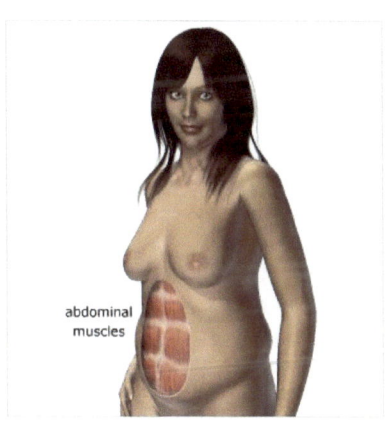

A way to test for it, is lie flat with your knees straight, raise the ankles off the bed and feel if there's a gap between your muscles, the gap may be on the upper part around the tummy muscle or the lower part. If there's a gap you will feel a pouch between the muscle or a gap between the muscle.

* Diastasis means splitting of the rectus(abdominal) muscles.

Body Lift

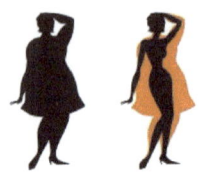
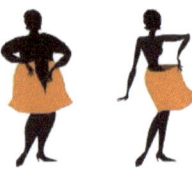

A body lift, also known as a lipectomy(or Beltectomy for back body lift), is a procedure to raise and reshape unsightly, sagging body contours. During the aging process and after weight loss, skin loses some elasticity, causing the mid-section to lose its natural shape and firmness. This procedure is designed to remove loose skin and related fat deposits, thus, providing a more youthful appearance. A body lift can be applied to the lower torso and upper legs including the abdomen, waist, inner/outer thighs, buttocks, and/or hips. Liposuction may also be completed in conjunction with a body lift.

Reasons for Considering a Body Lift:

• Reshape mid-body contour.
• Correct sagging skin and fat due to aging or excessive weight loss.
• Remedy weight gain and stretched skin caused by multiple pregnancies.

General Procedure

The precise procedure varies with each patient, depending on the body type and desired surgical outcome. Generally speaking, the body lift procedure entails making an incision that follows the upper and/or inner thigh, to the waistline. In more extensive surgeries, the incision goes completely around the waist and lower back.

Adjustments to the buttocks and thighs require an incision at the crease of the buttocks. Excess skin is then removed, followed by the underlying fat deposits. Finally, the skin is pulled taught and sutured into the new configuration. The entire procedure can last a few hours. The surgery is performed under general anesthesia.

Body Contouring

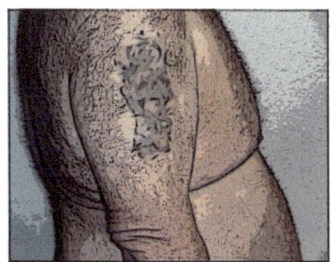

Body contouring after major weight loss reduces the excess skin and fat that is left behind from the expansion of skin, loss of fat and lack of tissue elasticity that often occurs after a major weight loss. This sagging skin commonly develops around the face, neck, upper arms, breast, abdomen, buttocks, and thighs and can make your body contour appear irregular and misshapen. If you have undergone dramatic weight loss either through diet and exercise or bariatric surgery, and you are at your optimum weight loss goal, you may be a good candidate for this surgery and may wish to consider undergoing this procedure.

Women who have lost large amounts of weight may find their breast has flattened and now sagged significantly. Body Contouring after major weight loss is an important and rewarding phase of your progress to a healthier more proportionate body and can help you to further enhance your body image and self confidence.

In general, surgical Body Contouring following major weight loss improves the shape and tone of the underlying tissue and removes excess fat and skin. The result is a more normal appearance to body with smoother contours.

The success of body contouring, whether it is done to reduce, enlarge or lift, is influenced by your age and by the size, shape and skin tone of the area to be treated. Some contouring procedures leave only small, inconspicuous scars. More noticeable scars may result when surgical removal of fat and skin is necessary to achieve your desired result. Most patients find these scars

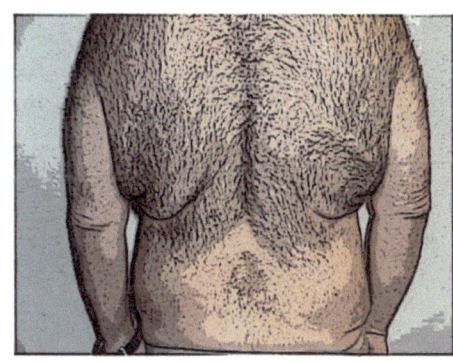

acceptable and enjoy greater self-confidence when wearing a bathing suit or form-fitting clothes.

Body Lift/Contouring Recovery Process

Generally, post-operative instructions require plenty of rest and limited movement in order to speed up the healing process and recovery time. Bandages are applied right after surgery to minimize swelling and provide support. Tubes are often placed to drain excess fluids. The scars resulting from the incisions are permanent but are carefully placed so as to minimize visibility. Patients

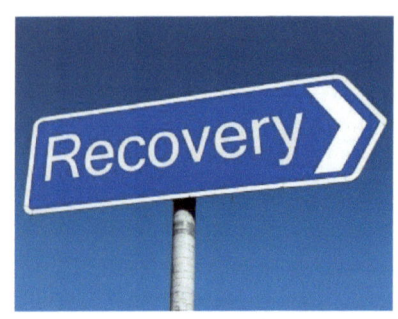

sometimes report minor pain associated with surgery which can be treated with oral medication. Recovery time varies with the extent of the procedure. While complications are rare, patients can minimize potential problems by carefully following the directions that are given after the surgery.

Please read our chapter on recovery instructions under "Frequently Asked Questions" for more information.

Corset Trunkplasty

The *Corset Trunkplasty is a comprehensive body contouring technique for patients following massive weight loss. The procedure addresses redundant skin of the entire abdomen, from the breastbone down to the pelvis, and provides an aesthetically pleasing full-length waistline.

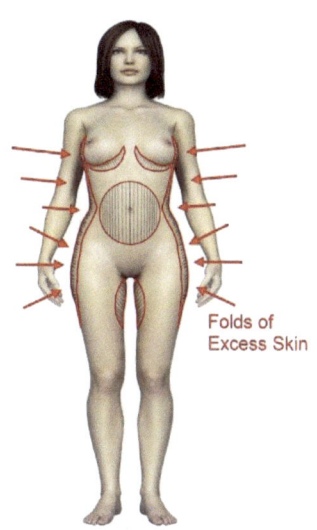

Folds of Excess Skin

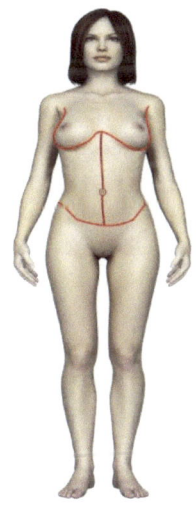

Corset Trunkplasty is a one step body contouring procedure for massive weight loss patients. It combines a Feur de-lis procedure with a reverse abdominoplasty. This will dramatically shape the abdomen and remove excess skin from the abdomen, axilla and hips. This will pull the patients anterior lateral skin tight(imagine pulling a corset very tight) and give curves and shape to patients who previously didn't have them.

*Dr Okpaku is one of a few surgeons in the country actively doing this procedure in addition to other post massive weight loss surgery. This is an outpatient surgery.

Lower Body Lift

A Lower Body Lift combines the Tummy Tuck Abdominoplasty sculpture of the stomach, with Thigh Lift, and Buttock Lift sculpting the entire body in a band about the waist or a Belt Lipectomy.

Excess skin and fat are removed, the stomach muscle wall tightened, and the Superficial Fascia Suspension System (SFS) resuspended. This connective tissue network in the fat contributes greatly to holding tissues elevated. The tone of this SFS is what gives a more youthful appearance and support to the entire sculpture. Liposuction is often combined with Body Lift Surgery to refine nearby regions of localized fat.

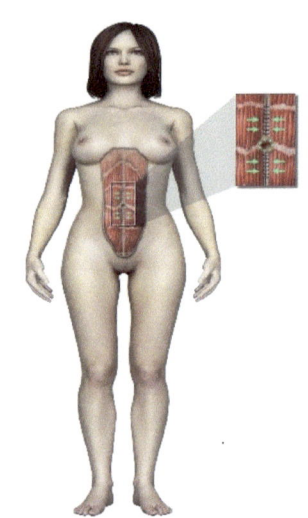

Body Lift Surgery is Not a Weight Loss Tool

Body Lift Surgery is a resuspension sculpture. It is not a alternative to losing weight or a motivational tool. Losing weight is a coarse tool. You cannot predict where the fat will come from. Plastic Surgery is better as a refinement tool. Major weight loss after Body Lift can result in further tissue sagging.

Removing Excess Residual Fat

In addition, even though the patient might have experienced massive weight reduction, this weight loss may not be evenly spread around the body. This also depends on the patient's type of obesity condition (whether gynoid or android). Bariatric plastic surgery procedures can help to reduce these fat deposits, either by surgical excision, body contouring or lipoplasty.

Lower Body Lift Procedure

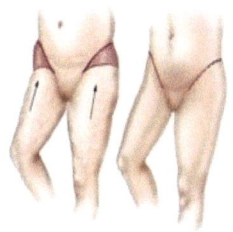 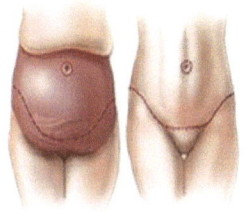 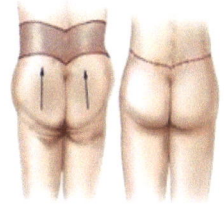

In one procedure, the sagging skin of the abdomen, outer thighs, buttocks, hips, and waist is corrected. Incisions extend completely around the body to remove a "belt" of excess skin and fat. Another common name for this procedure is a "belt lipectomy."

When people gain a lot of weight they usually deposit their fat around their entire lower trunk, which involves the front, sides and back starting from just below the ribs to the pelvic region. When they lose the weight they end up with folds of excess fat and skin that is most obvious in the front, often looking like an apron that will hang to varying degrees. However the hanging excess does not stop in the front, and most often it will continue on to the sides and the back involving the outer thighs, lower back, and buttocks regions. This type of problem is called circumferential excess.

To treat circumferential excess of the lower trunk in the massive weight loss patient, a lower body lift/belt lipectomy is most often employed. In this procedure, a wedge of tissue that goes around the lower aspect of the lower trunk is removed to treat the entire region so that the greatest amount of improvement can be attained. Although a tummy tuck/abdominoplasty, a procedure where only the front of the belly area is reduced, can be used in some massive weight loss patients, the results are often less than ideal because the sides and back are not adequately addressed.

Although these types of procedures are most often utilized in massive weight loss patients, there are three other groups that may benefit from this type of surgery:

- Women who were never obese but are 30 to 40 pounds overweight and are not able to lose the weight
- Patients who underwent liposuction with excess skin in the area of the lower trunk and/or thighs

Lower Body Lift Standard Procedure Techniques

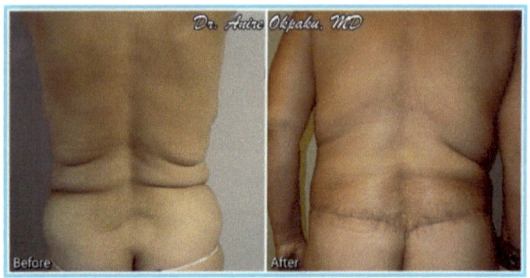

Lower Body Lift surgery involves removing a circumferential wedge of tissue. In the front the procedure involves removing the hanging apron of skin and fat and tightening up the underlying muscle wall, which is very similar to what is accomplished in a tummy tuck. To remove the excess tissues located in the back and sides the patient has to be turned in the operating room to allow for exposure of these areas. Liposuction of the thighs is often performed at the same time. The final scar has a similar shape to a "thong bikini" for most surgeons.

Lower Body Lift Recovery Process

• Patient must ambulate(walk) the day of surgery to help reduce chances of blood clots in legs

• This procedure may take 1 to 4 weeks to recover from

• Some surgeons prefer to use compression garments

• Most patients may be instructed to walk bent at the waist for a week

• Usually patients will have drains, plastic tubes that drain blood and body fluids, from the areas that were operated on. They will stay in place for a variable amount of time, from a few days to weeks

• The final results may not be apparent until all swelling has resolved which may take up to a year for this type of procedure

Surgery after massive weight loss should be thought of as an extensive operation and a major life event. Potential risk and complications may include:

- Bleeding, Infection
- Moderate to high potential for revisionary procedures
- Unattractive scarring
- Seroma formation, which are fluid collections that can arise after surgery along the operating site
- Separation of the incision because of the tension created by taking out the wedge of tissue
- Potential for blood clots in the legs (Deep Vein Thrombosis) that can travel to the lungs (pulmonary embolism)
- Difficulty in healing the incision edges together
- Death

FEATURED POST BARIATRIC SURGICAL PROCEDURE:

Dr. Okpaku's Total Body Lift™

Dr. Okpaku performs a new, cutting edge procedure which will greatly speed up recovery and improve on weight loss patient's overall appearance. Currently, patients who have lost 100-200 lbs or sometimes more weight, undergo three to five surgeries to remove the extra sagging skin. Some patients can have upwards of 30-50 lbs of skin removed during these surgeries. Some doctors were able to reduce the number of surgeries to 2-3 while still requiring multiple procedures.

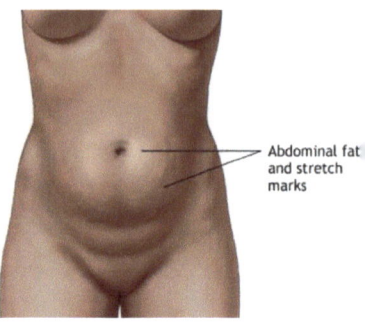

Abdominal fat and stretch marks

Traditional surgeries can take up to 8 hours or more per procedure.

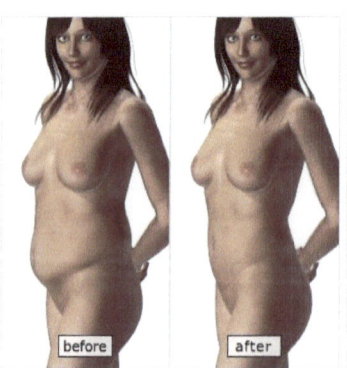

before

after

One current procedure used is called Corset Trunkplasty. The advantages of this surgery is that is cinches the waist tighter than the traditional Abdominoplasty(horizontal direction). It also reduces the redundant tissue from under the axilla region (armpit/bra roll). This gives the patient a much better look/shape of the waist, flanks and lower chest/armpit area than the traditional type of surgeries.

A traditional lower body lift requires many surgeries as the posterior(back) area is not done at the same time and usually takes between 6 to 8 hours to complete. The medial thigh lift, arm lift, breast reduction or breast lift are also commonly done as separate surgeries. In contrast, the **Okpaku Total Body Lift™** combines four different surgical procedures in a much shorter time period.

About The Okpaku Total Body Lift™

This combines the following procedures: Fleur de lis abdominoplasty, reverse (****fleur de lis**) abdominoplasty, axillary resection and beltectomy. By combining the four procedures we take the Corset Trunkplasty procedure and advance it further. This is also done in a shorter time period than the commonly performed body lift. Doing the procedure in less time than the standard treatments decreases certain complications commonly seen in this type of surgery.

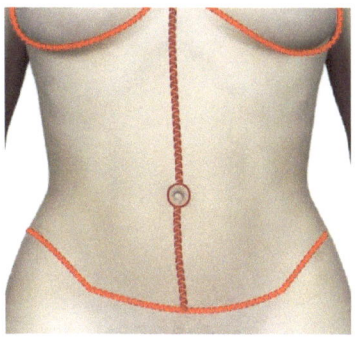

Dr. Okpaku utilizes the "**Harmonic Scalpel™**" technology for all body lift procedures. The Harmonic Scalpel™ helps to dramatically reduce the healing time. This new tool helps reduce seroma formations and need for drains (which are a leading complaints with post bariatric rehabilitation surgery). The patients also tend to have less intense pain after using the Harmonic instruments.

***The inverted T type or the **fleur de lis abdominoplasty** is suitable for the massive weight loss patients with midline abdominal scars or hernias. Open gastric bypass surgery often results in large post op. ventral hernias which need repair. Dermolipectomy and hernia repair with or without a mesh can be done simultaneously.*

The surgery is outpatient surgery, so the patient will be walking and eating and at home the same day of surgery. The drains will be removed in approximately one week after surgery. The patient will return to work generally in a week to 10 days. Traditional methods usually require 2 weeks off from work and drains could last a month or so, therefore the patient can more easily afford the surgery due to decrease time off of work and decreased surgery expenses.

"The brachioplasty and medial thigh lift are usually done in a separate operation. A facelift and/or breast reduction/mastopexy +/- breast augmentation can be performed at the same time the Okpaku Total Body Lift™ is performed, due to efficient use of operating room time. Instead of taking 3-5 surgeries which many surgeons typically perform, the patient is finished after typically 1-2 surgeries. This means less time off of work, less financial costs and less surgeries for the patients. In closing the Okpaku Total Body Lift™ has many advantages over the traditional post extreme weight lose surgery. It is a safer surgery, provides a better shape, quicker recovery, less time off of work, less expenses and less surgical procedures than the traditional method."

– Dr. Anire Okpaku, MD, FACS

Minimizing Scars

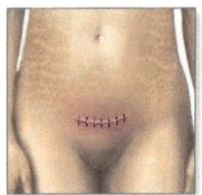 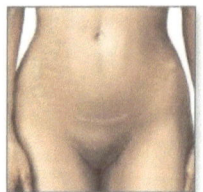

Whenever your skin gets cut, there will be scarring. Something as simple as skinning your knee may result in a scar. The same is true of cosmetic surgery, making an incision in the skin, which typically requires cutting through all of the layers of the skin, can result in scarring, regardless of where on the body surgery is performed. Furthermore, if you are currently overweight, you may be at greater risk for scarring. Why? The fat under your skin can work against our best efforts to close your incision seamlessly. Of course, surgery performed by a skilled surgeon results in a lesser degree of scarring, but many times the skill of the surgeon has only a small effect on the amount of scarring that takes place. A surgeon pays a great deal of attention to precisely close the incisions in a manner that minimizes scarring as much as possible. Keep in mind there are other factors beyond the surgeon's control that determine how badly you will scar.

There are certain factors beyond your control to influence your ability to heal without scarring. Although these risk factors cannot be changed, knowing them will help determine if you might scar badly after your procedure.

Risk Factors For Scarring:

- **Age**: As we age, our skin becomes less elastic and becomes thinner. This is because collagen (which makes the skin elastic) changes as we age, and the fat layer under our skin becomes thinner. The result of these changes, along with sun exposure, smoking, exposure to the environment and other lifestyle issues, means that skin does not heal as well or as quickly as we age. The benefit to age is that the imperfections that occur over time, like sun damage, work to help conceal scars that might be more obvious on younger skin.

- **Race**: Some races are more likely to scar than others. Black people are more likely to form hypertrophic, or keloid scars, which are an overgrowth of scar tissue at the site of an injury. Fair skinned people may find that their scars are more obvious than they would be with a darker complexion.

- **Inherited Tendency To Scar**: If your parents or siblings tend to scar heavily, you are likely to do the same. If you have a family tendency to scar badly, you should discuss this with your surgeon.

- **Size and Depth of Your Incision**: A large incision is much more likely to leave a scar than a small incision. The deeper and longer the incision, the longer the healing process will take and the greater the opportunity for scarring. A larger incision may be exposed to more stress as you move, which can cause slower healing.

- **How Quickly Your Skin Heals**: You may be one of the genetically blessed people who seem to heal magically, quickly and easily with minimal scarring, or you may be diabetic and your skin tends to heal slowly. How quickly you heal is a personal thing and can change with illness or injury.

Preparing for surgery: Some steps are simple, like following the instructions Dr. Okpaku gives you to the letter, yet others like quitting smoking will require a bigger effort.

- **Smoking**: Not only does smoking increase your risk for scars, it can also slow your healing. Smoking is such a significant risk factor that many plastic surgeons will not operate on a patient if he/she does not quit smoking COMPLETELY prior to surgery.

- **Drinking**: Alcohol dehydrates both the body and skin, which decreases your overall state of health. While your wound is healing, avoid alcohol and focus on non-caffeinated beverages.

- **Nutrition**: Eat a balanced diet with an emphasis on protein intake. Protein makes up the building blocks of healing skin, so it is essential to provide your body with adequate protein (chicken, pork, fish, seafood, beef, dairy products) to allow your skin to heal. If you do not like eating meat, soy products provide an excellent alternative as a lean protein source.

- **Hydration**: Dehydration happens when you are not taking in enough fluids. In severe cases, this can cause electrolyte imbalances and heart issues. In less severe cases, you will feel thirsty and your overall health will be diminished. Staying well hydrated (Tip: If you are well-hydrated, your urine will be almost colorless or light in color) will help keep your healing headed in the right direction.

- **Limit motion or tension on the scar:** This is particularly valuable in the first 6 weeks. Common locations of tension include the knees, back and neck.

- **Avoid sun/ UV rays:** This tends to pigment maturing scars. Protect with SPF 15 or higher for at least 1 year after surgery

- **Antibiotic ointment:** (such as Neosporin, Bacitracin, Triple antibiotic ointment) – Studies have shown that moist wound healing is quicker and results in better scars. Antibiotic ointment helps to hydrate the wound with the added benefit of decreasing bacteria in dirty wounds. Antibiotic ointment is beneficial when a wound in not completely healed (abrasion injury, cut, scrape, recently closed incision). This is recommended within the first 24-48 hours of a surgically repaired wound.

- **Use a Silicon product :** This helps to guard against scar formation after surgery or injury and flatten old raised scars. It is a fast-drying brush-on, clear liquid. Once dry, it is waterproof, nearly invisible and can be covered by makeup. Silicone scar products such as gels and sheets, flattens and softens scars. Even the color improves from being very red to a more skin like color.

Pre-Operative Instructions – The following instructions should be followed closely except when overruled by specific procedural instructions.

Two Weeks Prior to Surgery

- NO ASPIRIN or medicines that contain aspirin* since it interferes with normal blood clotting.
- NO IBUPROFEN or medicines contain ibuprofen* as it interferes with blood clotting.
- Please DISCONTINUE ALL HERBAL MEDICATIONS* as many have side effects that could complicate a surgical procedure by inhibiting blood clotting, affecting blood pressure, or interfering with anesthetics.
- Please DISCONTINUE ALL DIET PILLS whether prescription, over-the-counter or herbal as many will interfere with anesthesia and can cause cardiovascular concerns.
- NO "MEGADOSES" OF VITAMIN E, but a multiple vitamin that contains E is just fine.
- NO SMOKING because nicotine reduces blood flow to the skin and can cause significant complications during healing.
- You may take Tylenol or generic forms of this drug. These do not interfere with blood clotting or healing.
- Start taking a multivitamin each day and Vitamin C (1000 to 1500 mg) a day and continue taking through your recovery. The healthier you are, the quicker your recovery will be.

One Week Prior to Surgery

- DO NOT take or drink any alcohol or drugs for one week prior to surgery and one week after surgery as these can interfere with anesthesia and affect blood clotting.
- If your skin tolerates, use a germ-inhibiting soap (anti-bacterial soap) for bathing, such as Dial, Safeguard, or Lever 2000 for at least the week before surgery.
- DO report any signs of cold, infection, boils, or pustules appearing before surgery.
- DO NOT take any cough or cold medications without permission.
- DO arrange for a responsible adult to drive you to and from the facility on the day of surgery, since you will not be allowed to leave on your own.
- DO arrange for a responsible individual to spend the first 24 hours with you, since you CANNOT be left alone.

Night Before Surgery & Morning of Surgery

- DO NOT EAT or DRINK anything (not even water) after midnight the night before your surgery. Also, no gum, candy, mints or coffee the morning of surgery. Do not sneak anything as this may endanger you.
- If you are on regular medications, please clear these with your surgeon.
- DO take a thorough shower with your germ-inhibiting soap the night before and the morning of surgery. Shampoo your hair the morning of surgery. This is to decrease the bacteria on the skin and thereby decrease the risk of infection.
- DO NOT apply any of the following to your skin, hair or face the morning of surgery: makeup, creams, lotions, hair gels, sprays, perfumes, powder, or deodorant. Using any of these products will add bacteria to the skin and increase the risk of infection.
- You may brush your teeth the morning of surgery but do not drink or eat anything.
- DO NOT wear contacts to surgery. If you do wear glasses, bring your eyeglass case.
- DO wear comfortable, loose-fitting clothes that do not have to be put on over your head. The best thing to wear home is a button-up top and pull on pants. You will want easy-to-slip-on flat shoes.
- DO NOT bring any valuables or wear any jewelry (no rings, earrings, chains, toe rings, other metal piercings or watches). We will need to tape wedding rings if worn.
- You must have an adult drive for you – to and from surgery. Please note that a cab or bus driver will not be allowed to take you home after surgery. On arrival, be sure we know your driver's name, phone numbers, and how we will be able to reach them.
- If you are not recovering at home, it is very important that the doctor's office has the number where you will be after surgery

NOTE: Scar Treatment (1 to 4 weeks after surgery), ask your doctor about scar creams and silicone sheeting – For on-line ordering, please go to: www.drobodies.com and click on Dr.O Products and then click on recovery aids

Diet After Weight Loss Surgery:

Post bariatric surgery patients are put on a preop regiment of nutritional supplements and medications to get them optimized for surgery, starting several weeks or months prior to the corrective surgery. Our preop diet is nutrionally complete. Also preop exercise is important to get the patient in the best shape for the surgery that they can reasonable be in.

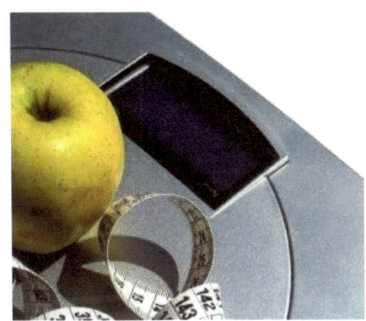

The following are Dr. Okpaku's guidelines for a very healthy diet:

1. Get rid of all the JUNK FOODS, poor nutritional foods and drinks in the house. Remove them and NEVER buy them again. Don't eat junk food.

2. Do not eat any products which are white ....i.e. white bread, crackers, pasta, rice, white potatoes, white sugar.

3. Do not eat 2 starches in one meal i.e. bread, crackers, pasta, rice, beans, starchy vegetables, etc.

4. NO FRIED FOODS!!! Only baked, broil or use a non stick pan to cook with. DO NOT add butter to food. Try not to add any oil when you cook. If you have to; only use olive or canola oil.

5. Drink lots of water (at least 48 oz). DO NOT DRINK sugar beverages. Limit drinking diet sodas (they can increase hunger). Limit drinking fruit juices (high in sugars and calories). You may drink home made vegetable juices. Vegetable juice is great for a snack and is low calories and is filling.

6. Serve yourself smaller portions. Use smaller plates and bowls. Meat portions should be under 4-5ozs which is about half your fist. Do not eat the skin of chicken and turkey etc. Pick meats with minimal fat and trim all the fat. Starches should be limited to one (1 serving) or less per meal. You can eat as much non-starchy vegetables as you want. Eat fruits.

7. Be careful of using salad dressings, ketchup and condiments. They can have large quantities of fat, sugars, preservatives, etc.

8. Read labels similar, foods made differently can have a massive difference in calories. DO NOT EAT foods with sugar or equivalent allowed such as, high fructose, corn syrup, sucrose, dextrose, etc.

9. Walk twice (2)a day for 20 minutes at a brisk pace. Work up to 30-40 minutes twice a day.

10. Drink a large glass of water 15-20 minutes or so before you eat.

"You need to commit to changing your life, only you can make it happen. Remember, if you fall of the wagon get back on it."
– Dr. Okpaku

Dr. Okpaku Questions & Answers:

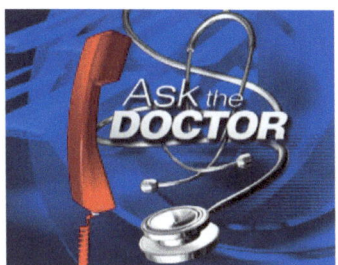

With the advent of the internet, there is now an array of information available for plastic surgery candidates to research. In addition, here we provide you with some common questions and answers on plastic surgery. If you have any other questions, and would like to contact us about it or would like to schedule an appointment, we would love to hear from you.

Q: Am I good candidate for lower body lift?

A: Lower Body Lift is indicated in patients who were obese and have lost a significant amount of weight leading to circumferential lower truncal excess. To operate on a patient they should:
be medically stable
be psychiatrically stable
have stabilized their weight loss (neither losing nor gaining weight)

Q: Is plastic surgery safe?

A: All surgical procedures are accompanied by a certain degree of risk, whether the procedures are for medical or cosmetic reasons. Our expert team is dedicated to making your operation go smoothly. We careful review your medical history and current health condition before deciding if it is safe for you to proceed with surgery. It is important that you fully disclose all pertinent information so that we are able to make an accurate assessment of the risks involved. We will take every precaution necessary to reduce the possibility of any complications.

Q: How do I know if plastic surgery is right for me?

A: There several important factors that come into play when deciding whether plastic surgery is the right option for you. One of the most important factors is your health. Being in good health greatly reduces the risk of complications occurring during surgery and leads to a speedy recovery. Next, you need to ask yourself what your motivations are. People who have plastic surgery generally find that the surgery enhances their overall appearance and self-esteem. You should have realistic expectations.

Plastic surgery is both a science and an art, neither of which are perfect.

Set reasonable goals as to the result you wish to achieve and be prepared to thoroughly discuss these goals during your initial consultation.

Q: Can I have several procedures performed simultaneously?

A: It is a relatively common practice for a plastic surgeon to perform multiple procedures during one operation. This allows the surgeon to better "sculpt" your final appearance. In addition, having several procedures done simultaneously saves you the expense of paying the operating room and anesthesia costs more than once. However, having too much done at one time can lead to complications. The decision to have multiple procedures done depends on which procedures are being done, the extent of surgery, the operating time, and your age/health. Ultimately, the surgeon decides whether or not it is appropriate to include more than one procedure in your operation.

Q: Does it matter how old I am?

A: Due to the variety of procedures available in plastic surgery, there can be no blanket rule on age although age will be taken into consideration when planning your operation. People of all ages have taken advantage of the image-enhancement offered by plastic surgery. It is important to realize the limitations of plastic surgery. Plastic surgery cannot "fix" every situation or reverse the aging process. What is a good procedure for one person may not be an appropriate procedure for another. We are committed to making your plastic surgery experience a successful one.

Q: What happens during my initial consultation?

A: During your consultation we will discuss your desired changes and expectations, review your medical history and current health, and make an assessment on whether the procedure(s) in question are right for you. This is a good time to ask specific questions about the procedure so that you are fully prepared, mentally and emotionally, for surgery. We will discuss the results that can be achieved, with the aid of photos and/or computer imaging. When a final decision is made, you will need to sign an informed consent stating that you are fully aware and understand what is entailed by your pending operation, including the potential complications and secondary effects.

Q: How long will it take to recover from my surgery?

A: Generally, post-operative instructions call for rest and limited movement in order to speed up the healing process and recovery time. The length of recovery varies with each procedure and is different for each individual. Bruises usually disappear within a few days, and most swelling is gone in a matter of weeks.

   If you follow our post-operative instructions carefully, you will be able to enjoy your normal activities within no time. Your scars will fade over time but are permanent. We take care to conceal any scars so that they are barely visible, if at all. The image-enhancing effects of plastic surgery become more evident over time.

It will take time for your body to fully adjust and settle into its new look. When you come in for your consultation we can discuss your expected recovery period and any post-operative instructions in detail.

Q: Will my insurance cover the surgery?

A: Insurance providers generally cover costs for reconstructive surgery but not for cosmetic surgery. For example, insurance providers will often pay for breast augmentation to reconstruct a breast following a mastectomy; breast reduction to remedy back pain caused by heavy breasts; eyelid surgery to remove sagging skin that blocks vision; nose surgery to allow for a patient to breathe better; or tummy tucks to remedy the vertical separation of abdomen muscles known as diastasis. Insurance providers are required by law to cover breast reconstruction surgery and any cosmetic operations necessary to create symmetry in either breast. If your surgery is covered by insurance, pre-certification is required.

Q: Will Arm Lift surgery be painful?

A:Postoperative pain is subjective and will vary considerably from person to person. The average patient undergoing an upper arm reduction procedure will usually require a few days of oral pain medication to treat discomfort. Over a 7 to 10 day period most people resolve the majority of their acute postoperative pain.

Q: Will there be scarring with Arm Lift surgery?

A: Upper arm reduction involves the removal of skin and necessitates the creation of a scar that starts near the elbow, traverses to the arm pit, and often crosses onto the chest wall. Any scar goes through a maturation process, which takes a year to complete. Most scars are conspicuous, at least initially. Some surgeons prefer to place the upper arm reduction scar on the inner arm aspect so that it is not visible when the patient's arm is by their side. Other surgeons prefer to place the scar a bit more towards the back of the arm so that it is not visible from the front, especially when the patient is observed from the front while moving the arm.

Q: What type of anesthesia will be used for Arm Lift surgery?

A: Most arm lifts are performed under a general anesthetic, although some surgeons will utilize a local anesthetic, with sedation. It is important that the facility that the procedure is performed in is an accredited facility where the type of anesthesia utilized is allowed.

About the author

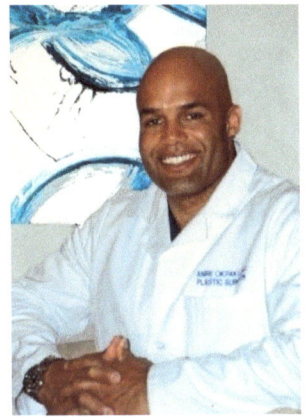

Doctor Anire Okpaku is a Board-Certified Plastic Surgeon and the Medical Director of Ocean View Plastic Surgery, serving the needs of Miami, Fort Lauderdale, and South Florida. He specializes in cosmetic plastic surgery.

He is an active member of the Bayside Medical Center at Mercy Hospital where he performs most of his surgeries. He also holds privileges in several other South Florida Hospitals.

Dr. Okpaku graduated from the prestigious Jefferson Medical College in Philadelphia, relocating later to Miami to where he completed his general surgical residency at Jackson Memorial Hospital University of Miami. He went on to complete a Plastic Surgery Fellowship at the University of Texas Health and Science Center, in San Antonio.

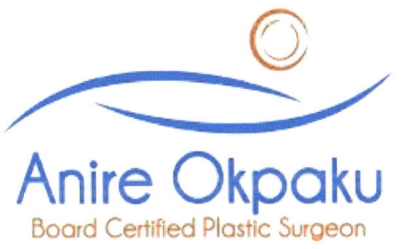

1900 Brickell Avenue
Miami, FL 33129
Phone : (305) 856-9566
Fax : (305) 856-9567
Site : www.DroBodies.com